INSTANT VORTEX

AIR FRYER

RECIPES

TASTY RECIPES FOR BEGINNERS

JAMES PENN

Table of Contents

Cauliflower, Chickpea, and Avocado Mash

Prep time: 10 minutes | Cook time: 25 minutes | Serves 4

1 medium head cauliflower, cut into florets

1 can chickpeas, drained and rinsed

1 tablespoon extra-virgin olive oil

2 tablespoons lemon juice

Salt and ground black pepper, to taste

4 flatbreads, toasted

2 ripe avocados, mashed

1. Set the temperature of the air fryer oven to 425ºF (218ºC). Press Start to begin preheating.

2. In a bowl, mix the chickpeas, cauliflower, lemon juice and olive oil. Sprinkle salt and pepper as desired.

3. Put inside the air fryer oven perforated pan and air fry for 25 minutes.

4. Spread on top of the flatbread along with the mashed avocado. Sprinkle with more pepper and salt and serve.

Cauliflower Faux Rice

Prep time: 15 minutes | Cook time: 40 minutes | Serves 8

1 large head cauliflower, rinsed and drained, cut into florets

½ lemon, juiced

2 garlic cloves, minced

2 (8-ounce / 227-g) cans mushrooms

1 (8-ounce / 227-g) can water chestnuts

¾ cup peas

1 egg, beaten

4 tablespoons soy sauce

1 tablespoon peanut oil

1 tablespoon sesame oil

1 tablespoon ginger, fresh and minced

Cooking spray

1. Set the temperature of the air fryer oven to 350ºF (177ºC). Press Start to begin preheating.

2. Mix the peanut oil, soy sauce, sesame oil, minced ginger, lemon juice, and minced garlic to combine well.

3. In a food processor, pulse the florets in small batches to break them down to resemble rice grains. Pour into the air fryer oven perforated pan.

4. Drain the can of water chestnuts and roughly chop them. Pour into the perforated pan. Air fry for 20 minutes.

5. In the meantime, drain the mushrooms. Add the mushrooms and the peas to the air fryer oven and continue to air fry for another 15 minutes.

6. Lightly spritz a frying pan with cooking spray. Prepare an omelet with the beaten egg, ensuring it is firm. Lay on a cutting board and slice it up.

7. When the cauliflower is ready, throw in the omelet and bake for an additional 5 minutes. Serve hot.

Chermoula Beet Roast

Prep time: 15 minutes | Cook time: 25 minutes | Serves 4

For the Chermoula:

1 cup packed fresh cilantro leaves

½ cup packed fresh parsley leaves

6 cloves garlic, peeled

2 teaspoons smoked paprika

2 teaspoons ground cumin

1 teaspoon ground coriander

½ to 1 teaspoon cayenne pepper

Pinch of crushed saffron (optional)

½ cup extra-virgin olive oil

Kosher salt, to taste

For the Beets:

3 medium beets, trimmed, peeled, and cut into 1-inch chunks

2 tablespoons chopped fresh cilantro

2 tablespoons chopped fresh parsley

1. In a food processor, combine the cilantro, parsley, garlic, paprika, cumin, coriander, and cayenne. Pulse until coarsely chopped. Add the saffron, if using, and process until combined. With the food processor running, slowly

add the olive oil in a steady stream; process until the sauce is uniform. Season with salt.

2. Set the temperature of the air fryer oven to 375ºF (191ºC). Press Start to begin preheating.

3. In a large bowl, drizzle the beets with ½ cup of the chermoula to coat. Arrange the beets in the air fryer oven perforated pan. Roast for 25 to minutes, or until the beets are tender.

4. Transfer the beets to a serving platter. Sprinkle with the chopped cilantro and parsley and serve.

Creamy and Cheesy Spinach

Prep time: 10 minutes | Cook time: 15 minutes | Serves 4

Vegetable oil spray

1 (10-ounce / 283-g) package frozen spinach, thawed and squeezed dry

½ cup chopped onion

2 cloves garlic, minced

4 ounces (113 g) cream cheese, diced

½ teaspoon ground nutmeg

1 teaspoon kosher salt

1 teaspoon black pepper

½ cup grated Parmesan cheese

1. Set the temperature of the air fryer oven to 350ºF (177ºC). Press Start to begin preheating. Spray a round heatproof pan with vegetable oil spray.

2. In a medium bowl, combine the spinach, onion, garlic, cream cheese, nutmeg, salt, and pepper. Transfer to the prepared pan.

3. Put the pan in the air fryer oven. Bake for 10 minutes. Open and stir to thoroughly combine the cream cheese and spinach.

4. Sprinkle the Parmesan cheese on top. Bake for 5 minutes, or until the cheese has melted and browned.

5. Serve hot.

Gold Ravioli

Prep time: 10 minutes | Cook time: 6 minutes | Serves 4

½ cup panko bread crumbs

2 teaspoons nutritional yeast

1 teaspoon dried basil

1 teaspoon dried oregano

1 teaspoon garlic powder

Salt and ground black pepper, to taste

¼ cup aquafaba

8 ounces (227 g) ravioli

Cooking spray

1. Cover the air fryer oven perforated pan with aluminum foil and coat with a light brushing of oil.

2. Set the temperature of the air fryer oven to 400ºF (204ºC). Press Start to begin preheating. Combine the panko bread crumbs, nutritional yeast, basil, oregano, and garlic powder. Sprinkle with salt and pepper to taste.

3. Put the aquafaba in a separate bowl. Dip the ravioli in the aquafaba before coating it in the panko mixture. Spritz with cooking spray and transfer to the air fryer oven.

4. Air fry for 6 minutes. Shake the air fryer oven perforated pan halfway.

5. Serve hot.

Green Beans with Shallot

Prep time: 10 minutes | Cook time: 10 minutes | Serves 4

1½ pounds (680 g) French green beans, stems removed and blanched

1 tablespoon salt

½ pound (227 g) shallots, peeled and cut into quarters

½ teaspoon ground white pepper

2 tablespoons olive oil

1. Set the temperature of the air fryer oven to 400ºF (204ºC). Press Start to begin preheating.

2. Coat the vegetables with the rest of the ingredients in a bowl.

3. Transfer to the perforated pan of the air fryer oven and air fry for 10 minutes, making sure the green beans achieve a light brown color.

4. Serve hot.

Lush Summer Rolls

Prep time: 15 minutes | Cook time: 15 minutes | Serves 4

1 cup shiitake mushroom, sliced thinly

1 celery stalk, chopped

1 medium carrot, shredded

½ teaspoon ginger, finely chopped

1 teaspoon sugar

1 tablespoon soy sauce

1 teaspoon nutritional yeast

8 spring roll sheets

1 teaspoon corn starch

2 tablespoons water

1. In a bowl, combine the ginger, soy sauce, nutritional yeast, carrots, celery, mushroom, and sugar.

2. Mix the cornstarch and water to create an adhesive for the spring rolls.

3. Scoop a tablespoonful of the vegetable mixture into the middle of the spring roll sheets. Brush the edges of the sheets with the cornstarch adhesive and enclose around the filling to make spring rolls.

4. Set the temperature of the air fryer oven to 400ºF (204ºC). Press Start to begin preheating. When warm, place the rolls inside and air fry for 15 minutes or until crisp.

5. Serve hot.

Lush Vegetables Roast

Prep time: 15 minutes | Cook time: 20 minutes | Serves 6

$1^1/_3$ cup small parsnips, peeled, cubed

$1\frac{1}{3}$ cup celery

2 red onions, sliced

$1\frac{1}{3}$ cup small butternut squash, cut in half, deseeded, cubed

1 tablespoon fresh thyme needles

1 tablespoon olive oil

Salt and ground black pepper, to taste

1. Set the temperature of the air fryer oven to 390ºF (199ºC). Press Start to begin preheating.

2. Combine the cut vegetables with the thyme, olive oil, salt and pepper.

3. Put the vegetables in the perforated pan and transfer the pan to the air fryer oven.

4. Roast for 20 minutes, stirring once throughout the roasting time, until the vegetables are nicely browned and cooked through.

5. Serve warm.

Mascarpone Mushrooms

Prep time: 10 minutes | Cook time: 15 minutes | Serves 4

Vegetable oil spray

4 cups sliced mushrooms

1 medium yellow onion, chopped

2 cloves garlic, minced

¼ cup heavy whipping cream or half-and-half

8 ounces (227 g) mascarpone cheese

1 teaspoon dried thyme

1 teaspoon kosher salt

1 teaspoon black pepper

½ teaspoon red pepper flakes

4 cups cooked konjac noodles, cauliflower rice, linguine, or spaghetti, for serving

½ cup grated Parmesan cheese

1. Set the temperature of the air fryer oven to 350ºF (177ºC). Press Start to begin preheating. Spray a round heatproof pan with vegetable oil spray.

2. In a medium bowl, combine the mushrooms, onion, garlic, cream, mascarpone, thyme, salt, black pepper, and red pepper flakes. Stir to combine. Transfer the mixture to the prepared pan.

3. Put the pan in the air fryer oven. Bake for 15 minutes, stirring halfway through the baking time.

4. Divide the pasta among four shallow bowls. Spoon the mushroom mixture evenly over the pasta. Sprinkle with Parmesan cheese and serve.

Mediterranean Air Fried Veggies

Prep time: 10 minutes | Cook time: 6 minutes | Serves 4

1 large zucchini, sliced

1 cup cherry tomatoes, halved

1 parsnip, sliced

1 green pepper, sliced

1 carrot, sliced

1 teaspoon mixed herbs

1 teaspoon mustard

1 teaspoon garlic purée

6 tablespoons olive oil

Salt and ground black pepper, to taste

1. Set the temperature of the air fryer oven to 400ºF (204ºC). Press Start to begin preheating.

2. Combine all the ingredients in a bowl, making sure to coat the vegetables well.

3. Transfer to the air fryer oven and air fry for 6 minutes, ensuring the vegetables are tender and browned.

4. Serve immediately.

Mushroom and Pepper Pizza Squares

Prep time: 10 minutes | Cook time: 10 minutes | Serves 10

1 pizza dough, cut into squares

1 cup oyster mushrooms, chopped

1 shallot, chopped

¼ red bell pepper, chopped

2 tablespoons parsley

Salt and ground black pepper, to taste

1. Set the temperature of the air fryer oven to 400ºF (204ºC). Press Start to begin preheating.

2. In a bowl, combine the oyster mushrooms, shallot, bell pepper and parsley. Sprinkle some salt and pepper as desired.

3. Spread this mixture on top of the pizza squares.

4. Bake in the air fryer oven for 10 minutes.

5. Serve warm.

Potato and Broccoli with Tofu Scramble

Prep time: 15 minutes | Cook time: 30 minutes | Serves 3

2½ cups chopped red potato

2 tablespoons olive oil, divided

1 block tofu, chopped finely

2 tablespoons tamari

1 teaspoon turmeric powder

½ teaspoon onion powder

½ teaspoon garlic powder

½ cup chopped onion

4 cups broccoli florets

1. Set the temperature of the air fryer oven to 400ºF (204ºC). Press Start to begin preheating.

2. Toss together the potatoes and 1 tablespoon of olive oil.

3. Air fry the potatoes in a baking dish for 15 minutes, shaking once during the cooking time to ensure they fry evenly.

4. Combine the tofu, remaining olive oil, turmeric, onion powder, tamari, and garlic powder together, before stirring in the onions, followed by the broccoli.

5. Top the potatoes with the tofu mixture and air fry for an additional 15 minutes. Serve warm.

Potatoes with Zucchinis

Prep time: 10 minutes | Cook time: 45 minutes | Serves 4

2 potatoes, peeled and cubed

4 carrots, cut into chunks

1 head broccoli, cut into florets

4 zucchinis, sliced thickly

Salt and ground black pepper, to taste

¼ cup olive oil

1 tablespoon dry onion powder

1. Set the temperature of the air fryer oven to 400ºF (204ºC). Press Start to begin preheating.

2. In a baking dish, add all the ingredients and combine well.

3. Bake for 45 minutes in the air fryer oven, ensuring the vegetables are soft and the sides have browned before serving.

Ratatouille

Prep time: 20 minutes | Cook time: 25 minutes | Serves 4

1 sprig basil

1 sprig flat-leaf parsley

1 sprig mint

1 tablespoon coriander powder

1 teaspoon capers

½ lemon, juiced

Salt and ground black pepper, to taste

2 eggplants, sliced crosswise

2 red onions, chopped

4 cloves garlic, minced

2 red peppers, sliced crosswise

1 fennel bulb, sliced crosswise

3 large zucchinis, sliced crosswise

5 tablespoons olive oil

4 large tomatoes, chopped

2 teaspoons herbs de Provence

1. Blend the basil, parsley, coriander, mint, lemon juice and capers, with a little salt and pepper. Make sure all ingredients are well-incorporated.

2. Set the temperature of the air fryer oven to 400ºF (204ºC). Press Start to begin preheating.

3. Coat the eggplant, onions, garlic, peppers, fennel, and zucchini with olive oil.

4. Take a baking dish small enough to fit inside the air fryer oven. Transfer the vegetables into a baking dish and top with the tomatoes and herb purée. Sprinkle with more salt and pepper, and the herbs de Provence.

5. Air fry for 25 minutes.

6. Serve immediately.

Rice and Eggplant Bowl

Prep time: 15 minutes | Cook time: 10 minutes | Serves 4

¼ cup sliced cucumber

1 teaspoon salt

1 tablespoon sugar

7 tablespoons Japanese rice vinegar

3 medium eggplants, sliced

3 tablespoons sweet white miso paste

1 tablespoon mirin rice wine

4 cups cooked sushi rice

4 spring onions

1 tablespoon toasted sesame seeds

1. Coat the cucumber slices with the rice wine vinegar, salt, and sugar.

2. Put a dish on top of the bowl to weight it down completely.

3. In a bowl, mix the eggplants, mirin rice wine, and miso paste. Allow to marinate for half an hour.

4. Set the temperature of the air fryer oven to 400ºF (204ºC). Press Start to begin preheating.

5. Put the eggplant slices in the air fryer oven and air fry for 10 minutes.

6. Fill the bottom of a serving bowl with rice and top with the eggplants and pickled cucumbers.

7. Add the spring onions and sesame seeds for garnish. Serve immediately.

Russet Potato Gratin

Prep time: 10 minutes | Cook time: 35 minutes | Serves 6

½ cup milk

7 medium russet potatoes, peeled

Salt, to taste

1 teaspoon black pepper

½ cup heavy whipping cream

½ cup grated semi-mature cheese

½ teaspoon nutmeg

1. Set the temperature of the air fryer oven to 390ºF (199ºC). Press Start to begin preheating.

2. Cut the potatoes into wafer-thin slices.

3. In a bowl, combine the milk and cream and sprinkle with salt, pepper, and nutmeg.

4. Use the milk mixture to coat the slices of potatoes. Put in a baking dish. Top the potatoes with the rest of the milk mixture.

5. Put the baking dish into the perforated pan of the air fryer oven and bake for 25 minutes.

6. Pour the cheese over the potatoes.

7. Bake for an additional 10 minutes, ensuring the top is nicely browned before serving.

Spicy Cauliflower Roast

Prep time: 15 minutes | Cook time: 20 minutes | Serves 4

For the Cauliflower:

5 cups cauliflower florets

3 tablespoons vegetable oil

½ teaspoon ground cumin

½ teaspoon ground coriander

½ teaspoon kosher salt

For the Sauce:

½ cup Greek yogurt or sour cream

¼ cup chopped fresh cilantro

1 jalapeño, coarsely chopped

4 cloves garlic, peeled

½ teaspoon kosher salt

2 tablespoons water

1. Set the temperature of the air fryer oven to 400ºF (204ºC). Press Start to begin preheating.

2. In a large bowl, combine the cauliflower, oil, cumin, coriander, and salt. Toss to coat.

3. Put the cauliflower in the air fryer oven perforated pan. Roast for 20 minutes, stirring halfway through the roasting time.

4. Meanwhile, in a blender, combine the yogurt, cilantro, jalapeño, garlic, and salt. Blend, adding the water as needed to keep the blades moving and to thin the sauce.

5. At the end of roasting time, transfer the cauliflower to a large serving bowl. Pour the sauce over and toss gently to coat. Serve immediately.

Super Vegetable Burger

Prep time: 15 minutes | Cook time: 12 minutes | Serves 8

½ pound (227 g) cauliflower, steamed and diced, rinsed and drained

2 teaspoons coconut oil, melted

2 teaspoons minced garlic

¼ cup desiccated coconut

½ cup oats

3 tablespoons flour

1 tablespoon flaxseeds plus 3 tablespoons water, divided

1 teaspoon mustard powder

2 teaspoons thyme

2 teaspoons parsley

2 teaspoons chives

Salt and ground black pepper, to taste

1 cup bread crumbs

1. Set the temperature of the air fryer oven to 390ºF (199ºC). Press Start to begin preheating.

2. Combine the cauliflower with all the ingredients, except for the bread crumbs, incorporating everything well.

3. Using the hands, shape 8 equal-sized amounts of the mixture into burger patties. Coat the patties in bread crumbs before putting them in the air fryer oven perforated pan in a single layer.

4. Air fry for 12 minutes or until crispy.

5. Serve hot.

Super Veg Rolls

Prep time: 20 minutes | Cook time: 10 minutes | Serves 6

2 potatoes, mashed

¼ cup peas

¼ cup mashed carrots

1 small cabbage, sliced

¼ cup beans

2 tablespoons sweetcorn

1 small onion, chopped

½ cup bread crumbs

1 packet spring roll sheets

½ cup cornstarch slurry

1. Set the temperature of the air fryer oven to 390ºF (199ºC). Press Start to begin preheating.

2. Boil all the vegetables in water over a low heat. Rinse and allow to dry.

3. Unroll the spring roll sheets and spoon equal amounts of vegetable onto the center of each one. Fold into spring rolls and coat each one with the slurry and bread crumbs.

4. Air fry the rolls in the preheated air fryer oven for 10 minutes.

5. Serve warm.

Sweet Potatoes with Tofu

Prep time: 15 minutes | Cook time: 35 minutes | Serves 8

8 sweet potatoes, scrubbed

2 tablespoons olive oil

1 large onion, chopped

2 green chilies, deseeded and chopped

8 ounces (227 g) tofu, crumbled

2 tablespoons Cajun seasoning

1 cup tomatoes

1 can kidney beans, drained and rinsed

Salt and ground black pepper, to taste

1. Set the temperature of the air fryer oven to 400ºF (204ºC). Press Start to begin preheating.

2. With a knife, pierce the skin of the sweet potatoes and air fry in the air fryer oven for 30 minutes or until soft.

3. Remove from the air fryer oven, halve each potato, and set to one side.

4. Over a medium heat, fry the onions and chilies in the olive oil in a skillet for 2 minutes until fragrant.

5. Add the tofu and Cajun seasoning and air fry for a further 3 minutes before incorporating the kidney beans and tomatoes. Sprinkle some salt and pepper as desire.

6. Top each sweet potato halve with a spoonful of the tofu mixture and serve.

Sweet Potatoes with Zucchini

Prep time: 20 minutes | Cook time: 20 minutes | Serves 4

2 large-sized sweet potatoes, peeled and quartered

1 medium zucchini, sliced

1 Serrano pepper, deseeded and thinly sliced

1 bell pepper, deseeded and thinly sliced

1 to 2 carrots, cut into matchsticks

¼ cup olive oil

1½ tablespoons maple syrup

½ teaspoon porcini powder

¼ teaspoon mustard powder

½ teaspoon fennel seeds

1 tablespoon garlic powder

½ teaspoon fine sea salt

¼ teaspoon ground black pepper

Tomato ketchup, for serving

1. Put the sweet potatoes, zucchini, peppers, and the carrot into the perforated pan of the air fryer oven. Coat with a drizzling of olive oil.

2. Set the temperature of the air fryer oven to 350ºF (177ºC). Press Start to begin preheating.

3. Air fry the vegetables for 15 minutes.

4. In the meantime, prepare the sauce by vigorously combining the other ingredients, except for the tomato ketchup, with a whisk.

5. Lightly grease a baking dish small enough to fit inside the air fryer oven.

6. Transfer the cooked vegetables to the baking dish, pour over the sauce and coat the vegetables well.

7. Increase the temperature to 390ºF (199ºC) and air fry the vegetables for an additional 5 minutes.

8. Serve warm with a side of ketchup.

Air Fried Asparagus

Prep time: 5 minutes | Cook time: 5 minutes | Serves 4

1 pound (454 g) fresh asparagus spears, trimmed

1 tablespoon olive oil

Salt and ground black pepper, to taste

1. Set the temperature of the air fryer oven to 375ºF (191ºC). Press Start to begin preheating.
2. Combine all the ingredients and transfer to the air fryer oven.
3. Air fry for 5 minutes or until soft.
4. Serve hot.

Air Fried Brussels Sprout

Prep time: 5 minutes | Cook time: 10 minutes | Serves 1

1 pound (454 g) Brussels sprouts

1 tablespoon coconut oil, melted

1 tablespoon unsalted butter, melted

1. Set the temperature of the air fryer oven to 400ºF (204ºC). Press Start to begin preheating.

2. Prepare the Brussels sprouts by halving them, discarding any loose leaves.

3. Combine with the melted coconut oil and transfer to the air fryer oven perforated pan.

4. Air fry for 10 minutes, giving the perforated pan a good shake throughout the air frying time to brown them up if desired.

5. The sprouts are ready when they are partially caramelized. Remove them from the air fryer oven and serve with a topping of melted butter before serving.

Air Fried Potatoes with Olives

Prep time: 15 minutes | Cook time: 40 minutes | Serves 1

1 medium russet potato, scrubbed and peeled

1 teaspoon olive oil

¼ teaspoon onion powder

⅛ teaspoon salt

Dollop of butter

Dollop of cream cheese

1 tablespoon Kalamata olives

1 tablespoon chives, chopped

1. Set the temperature of the air fryer oven to 400ºF (204ºC). Press Start to begin preheating.

2. In a bowl, coat the potatoes with the onion powder, salt, olive oil, and butter.

3. Transfer to the air fryer oven and air fry for 40 minutes, turning the potatoes over at the halfway point.

4. Take care when removing the potatoes from the air fryer oven and serve with the cream cheese, Kalamata olives and chives on top.

Cauliflower Tater Tots

Prep time: 15 minutes | Cook time: 16 minutes | Serves 12

1 pound (454 g) cauliflower, steamed and chopped

½ cup nutritional yeast

1 tablespoon oats

1 tablespoon desiccated coconuts plus 3 tablespoons flaxseed meal plus 3 tablespoons water

1 onion, chopped

1 teaspoon garlic, minced

1 teaspoon parsley, chopped

1 teaspoon oregano, chopped

1 teaspoon chives, chopped

Salt and ground black pepper, to taste

½ cup bread crumbs

1. Set the temperature of the air fryer oven to 390ºF (199ºC). Press Start to begin preheating.

2. Drain any excess water out of the cauliflower by wringing it with a paper towel.

3. In a bowl, combine the cauliflower with the remaining ingredients, save the bread crumbs. Using the hands, shape the mixture into several small balls.

4. Coat the balls in the bread crumbs and transfer to the perforated pan of the air fryer oven. Air fry for 6 minutes, then raise the temperature to 400ºF (204ºC) and then air fry for an additional 10 minutes.

5. Serve immediately.

Cheesy Macaroni Balls

Prep time: 10 minutes | Cook time: 10 minutes | Serves 2

2 cups leftover macaroni

1 cup shredded Cheddar cheese

½ cup flour

1 cup bread crumbs

3 large eggs

1 cup milk

½ teaspoon salt

¼ teaspoon black pepper

1. Set the temperature of the air fryer oven to 365ºF (185ºC). Press Start to begin preheating.

2. In a bowl, combine the leftover macaroni and shredded cheese.

3. Pour the flour in a separate bowl. Put the bread crumbs in a third bowl. Finally, in a fourth bowl, mix the eggs and milk with a whisk.

4. With an ice-cream scoop, create balls from the macaroni mixture. Coat them the flour, then in the egg mixture, and lastly in the bread crumbs.

5. Arrange the balls in the preheated air fryer oven and air fry for about 10 minutes, giving them an occasional stir. Ensure they crisp up nicely.

6. Serve hot.

Chili Fingerling Potatoes

Prep time: 10 minutes | Cook time: 16 minutes | Serves 4

1 pound (454 g) fingerling potatoes, rinsed and cut into wedges

1 teaspoon olive oil

1 teaspoon salt

1 teaspoon black pepper

1 teaspoon cayenne pepper

1 teaspoon nutritional yeast

½ teaspoon garlic powder

1. Set the temperature of the air fryer oven to 400ºF (204ºC). Press Start to begin preheating.
2. Coat the potatoes with the rest of the ingredients.
3. Transfer to the perforated pan of the air fryer oven and air fry for 16 minutes, shaking the perforated pan at the halfway point.
4. Serve immediately.

Corn Pakodas

Prep time: 10 minutes | Cook time: 8 minutes | Serves 5

1 cup flour

¼ teaspoon baking soda

¼ teaspoon salt

½ teaspoon curry powder

½ teaspoon red chili powder

¼ teaspoon turmeric powder

¼ cup water

10 cobs baby corn, blanched

Cooking spray

1. Set the temperature of the air fryer oven to 425ºF (218ºC). Press Start to begin preheating.

2. Cover the air fryer oven perforated pan with aluminum foil and spritz with cooking spray.

3. In a bowl, combine all the ingredients save for the corn. Stir with a whisk until well combined.

4. Coat the corn in the batter and put in the perforated pan.

5. Air fry for 8 minutes until a golden brown color is achieved.

6. Serve hot.

Crispy Chickpeas

Prep time: 5 minutes | Cook time: 15 minutes | Serves 4

1 (15-ounces / 425-g) can chickpeas, drained but not rinsed

2 tablespoons olive oil

1 teaspoon salt

2 tablespoons lemon juice

1. Set the temperature of the air fryer oven to 400ºF (204ºC). Press Start to begin preheating.

2. Add all the ingredients together in a bowl and mix. Transfer this mixture to the perforated pan of the air fryer oven.

3. Air fry for 15 minutes, ensuring the chickpeas become nice and crispy.

4. Serve immediately.

Crispy Jicama Fries

Prep time: 5 minutes | Cook time: 20 minutes | Serves 1

1 small jicama, peeled

¼ teaspoon onion powder

¾ teaspoon chili powder

¼ teaspoon garlic powder

¼ teaspoon ground black pepper

1. Set the temperature of the air fryer oven to 350ºF (177ºC). Press Start to begin preheating.

2. To make the fries, cut the jicama into matchsticks of the desired thickness.

3. In a bowl, toss them with the onion powder, chili powder, garlic powder, and black pepper to coat. Transfer the fries into the perforated pan of the air fryer oven.

4. Air fry for 20 minutes, giving the perforated pan an occasional shake throughout the cooking process. The fries are ready when they are hot and golden.

5. Serve immediately.

Easy Potato Croquettes

Prep time: 15 minutes | Cook time: 15 minutes | Serves 10

¼ cup nutritional yeast

2 cups boiled potatoes, mashed

1 flax egg (1 tablespoon flaxseed meal plus 3 tablespoons water)

1 tablespoon flour

2 tablespoons chives, chopped

Salt and ground black pepper, to taste

2 tablespoons vegetable oil

¼ cup bread crumbs

1. Set the temperature of the air fryer oven to 400ºF (204ºC). Press Start to begin preheating.

2. In a bowl, combine the nutritional yeast, potatoes, flax egg, flour, and chives. Sprinkle with salt and pepper as desired.

3. In a separate bowl, mix the vegetable oil and bread crumbs to achieve a crumbly consistency.

4. Shape the potato mixture into small balls and dip each one into the bread crumb mixture.

5. Put the croquettes inside the air fryer oven and air fry for 15 minutes, ensuring the croquettes turn golden brown.

6. Serve immediately.

Easy Rosemary Green Beans

Prep time: 5 minutes | Cook time: 5 minutes | Serves 1

1 tablespoon butter, melted

2 tablespoons rosemary

½ teaspoon salt

3 cloves garlic, minced

¾ cup green beans, chopped

1. Set the temperature of the air fryer oven to 390ºF (199ºC). Press Start to begin preheating.
2. Combine the melted butter with the rosemary, salt, and minced garlic. Toss in the green beans, coating them well.
3. Air fry for 5 minutes.
4. Serve immediately.

Fig, Chickpea, and Arugula Salad

Prep time: 15 minutes | Cook time: 20 minutes | Serves 4

8 fresh figs, halved

1½ cups chickpeas, cooked

1 teaspoon cumin seeds, roasted, crushed

4 tablespoons balsamic vinegar

2 tablespoons extra-virgin olive oil, plus more for greasing

Salt and ground black pepper, to taste

3 cups arugula rocket, washed and dried

1. Set the temperature of the air fryer oven to 375ºF (191ºC). Press Start to begin preheating.

2. Cover the air fryer oven perforated pan with aluminum foil and grease lightly with oil. Put the figs in the perforated pan and air fry for 10 minutes.

3. In a bowl, combine the chickpeas and cumin seeds.

4. Remove the air fried figs from the air fryer oven and replace with the chickpeas. Air fry for 10 minutes. Leave to cool.

5. In the meantime, prepare the dressing. Mix the balsamic vinegar, olive oil, salt and pepper.

6. In a salad bowl combine the arugula rocket with the cooled figs and chickpeas.

7. Toss with the sauce and serve.

Golden Pickles

Prep time: 10 minutes | Cook time: 15 minutes | Serves 4

14 dill pickles, sliced

¼ cup flour

⅛ teaspoon baking powder

Pinch of salt

2 tablespoons cornstarch plus 3 tablespoons water

6 tablespoons panko bread crumbs

½ teaspoon paprika

Cooking spray

1. Set the temperature of the air fryer oven to 400ºF (204ºC). Press Start to begin preheating.

2. Drain any excess moisture out of the dill pickles on a paper towel.

3. In a bowl, combine the flour, baking powder and salt.

4. Throw in the cornstarch and water mixture and combine well with a whisk.

5. Put the panko bread crumbs in a shallow dish along with the paprika. Mix thoroughly.

6. Dip the pickles in the flour batter, before coating in the bread crumbs. Spritz all the pickles with the cooking spray.

7. Transfer to the air fryer oven and air fry for 15 minutes, or until golden brown.

8. Serve immediately.

Herbed Radishes

Prep time: 5 minutes | Cook time: 10 minutes | Serves 2

1 pound (454 g) radishes

2 tablespoons unsalted butter, melted

¼ teaspoon dried oregano

½ teaspoon dried parsley

½ teaspoon garlic powder

1. Set the temperature of the air fryer oven to 350ºF (177ºC). Press Start to begin preheating. Prepare the radishes by cutting off their tops and bottoms and quartering them.

2. In a bowl, combine the butter, dried oregano, dried parsley, and garlic powder. Toss with the radishes to coat.

3. Transfer the radishes to the air fryer oven perforated pan and air fry for 10 minutes, shaking the perforated pan at the halfway point to ensure the radishes air fry evenly through. The radishes are ready when they turn brown.

4. Serve immediately.

Lemony Falafel

Prep time: 15 minutes | Cook time: 15 minutes | Serves 8

1 teaspoon cumin seeds

½ teaspoon coriander seeds

2 cups chickpeas, drained and rinsed

½ teaspoon red pepper flakes

3 cloves garlic

¼ cup parsley, chopped

¼ cup coriander, chopped

½ onion, diced

1 tablespoon juice from freshly squeezed lemon

3 tablespoons flour

½ teaspoon salt

Cooking spray

1. Fry the cumin and coriander seeds over medium heat until fragrant.

2. Grind using a mortar and pestle.

3. Put all of ingredients, except for the cooking spray, in a food processor and blend until a fine consistency is achieved.

4. Use the hands to mold the mixture into falafels and spritz with the cooking spray.

5. Set the temperature of the air fryer oven to 400ºF (204ºC). Press Start to begin preheating.

6. Transfer the falafels to the air fryer oven in one layer.

7. Air fry for 15 minutes, serving when they turn golden brown.

Lush Vegetable Salad

Prep time: 15 minutes | Cook time: 10 minutes | Serves 4

6 plum tomatoes, halved

2 large red onions, sliced

4 long red pepper, sliced

2 yellow pepper, sliced

6 cloves garlic, crushed

1 tablespoon extra-virgin olive oil

1 teaspoon paprika

½ lemon, juiced

Salt and ground black pepper, to taste

1 tablespoon baby capers

1. Set the temperature of the air fryer oven to 420ºF (216ºC). Press Start to begin preheating.

2. Put the tomatoes, onions, peppers, and garlic in a large bowl and cover with the extra-virgin olive oil, paprika, and lemon juice. Sprinkle with salt and pepper as desired.

3. Line the inside of the air fryer oven with aluminum foil. Put the vegetables inside and air fry for 10 minutes, ensuring the edges turn brown.

4. Serve in a salad bowl with the baby capers.

Potato with Creamy Cheese

Prep time: 5 minutes | Cook time: 15 minutes | Serves 2

2 medium potatoes

1 teaspoon butter

3 tablespoons sour cream

1 teaspoon chives

1½ tablespoons Parmesan cheese, grated

Salt and ground black pepper, to taste

1. Set the temperature of the air fryer oven to 350ºF (177ºC). Press Start to begin preheating.
2. Pierce the potatoes with a fork and boil them in water until they are cooked.
3. Transfer to the air fryer oven and air fry for 15 minutes.
4. In the meantime, combine the sour cream, cheese and chives in a bowl. Cut the potatoes halfway to open them up and fill with the butter and sour cream mixture.
5. Serve immediately.

Roasted Eggplant Slices

Prep time: 5 minutes | Cook time: 15 minutes | Serves 1

1 large eggplant, sliced

2 tablespoons olive oil

¼ teaspoon salt

½ teaspoon garlic powder

1. Set the temperature of the air fryer oven to 390ºF (199ºC). Press Start to begin preheating.

2. Apply the olive oil to the slices with a brush, coating both sides. Season each side with sprinklings of salt and garlic powder.

3. Put the slices in the air fryer oven and roast for 15 minutes.

4. Serve immediately.

Roasted Lemony Broccoli

Prep time: 5 minutes | Cook time: 15 minutes | Serves 6

2 heads broccoli, cut into florets

2 teaspoons extra-virgin olive oil, plus more for coating

1 teaspoon salt

½ teaspoon black pepper

1 clove garlic, minced

½ teaspoon lemon juice

1. Cover the air fryer oven perforated pan with aluminum foil and coat with a light brushing of oil.

2. Set the temperature of the air fryer oven to 375ºF (191ºC). Press Start to begin preheating.

3. In a bowl, combine all ingredients save for the lemon juice and transfer to the perforated pan. Roast for 15 minutes.

4. Serve with the lemon juice.

Roasted Potatoes and Asparagus

Prep time: 5 minutes | Cook time: 23 minutes | Serves 4

4 medium potatoes

1 bunch asparagus

⅓ cup cottage cheese

⅓ cup low-fat crème fraiche

1 tablespoon wholegrain mustard

Salt and pepper, to taste

Cook spray

1. Grease the perforated pan in the air fryer oven and set the temperature to 390ºF (199ºC). Press Start to begin preheating.

2. Air fry the potatoes in the air fryer oven for 20 minutes.

3. Boil the asparagus in salted water for 3 minutes.

4. Remove the potatoes and mash them with remaining ingredients. Sprinkle with salt and pepper.

5. Serve immediately.

Saltine Wax Beans

Prep time: 10 minutes | Cook time: 7 minutes | Serves 4

½ cup flour

1 teaspoon smoky chipotle powder

½ teaspoon ground black pepper

1 teaspoon sea salt flakes

2 eggs, beaten

½ cup crushed saltines

10 ounces (283 g) wax beans

Cooking spray

1. Set the temperature of the air fryer oven to 360ºF (182ºC). Press Start to begin preheating.

2. Combine the flour, chipotle powder, black pepper, and salt in a bowl. Put the eggs in a second bowl. Put the crushed saltines in a third bowl.

3. Wash the beans with cold water and discard any tough strings.

4. Coat the beans with the flour mixture, before dipping them into the beaten egg. Cover them with the crushed saltines.

5. Spritz the beans with cooking spray.

6. Air fry in the perforated pan of the air fryer oven for 4 minutes. Give the perforated pan a good shake and continue to air fry for 3 minutes. Serve hot.

Sesame Taj Tofu

Prep time: 5 minutes | Cook time: 25 minutes | Serves 4

1 block firm tofu, pressed and cut into 1-inch thick cubes

2 tablespoons soy sauce

2 teaspoons sesame seeds, toasted

1 teaspoon rice vinegar

1 tablespoon cornstarch

1. Set the temperature of the air fryer oven to 400ºF (204ºC). Press Start to begin preheating.

2. Add the tofu, soy sauce, sesame seeds, and rice vinegar in a bowl together and mix well to coat the tofu cubes. Then cover the tofu in cornstarch and put it in the perforated pan of the air fryer oven.

3. Air fry for 25 minutes, giving the perforated pan a shake at five-minute intervals to ensure the tofu cooks evenly.

4. Serve immediately.

Simple Buffalo Cauliflower

Prep time: 5 minutes | Cook time: 5 minutes | Serves 1

½ packet dry ranch seasoning

2 tablespoons salted butter, melted

1 cup cauliflower florets

¼ cup buffalo sauce

1. Set the temperature of the air fryer oven to 400ºF (204ºC). Press Start to begin preheating.

2. In a bowl, combine the dry ranch seasoning and butter. Toss with the cauliflower florets to coat and transfer them to the air fryer oven.

3. Roast for 5 minutes, shaking the perforated pan occasionally to ensure the florets roast evenly.

4. Remove the cauliflower from the air fryer oven, pour the buffalo sauce over it, and serve.

Simple Pesto Gnocchi

Prep time: 10 minutes | Cook time: 15 minutes | Serves 4

1 (1-pound / 454-g) package gnocchi

1 medium onion, chopped

3 cloves garlic, minced

1 tablespoon extra-virgin olive oil

1 (8-ounce / 227-g) jar pesto

⅓ cup grated Parmesan cheese

1. Set the temperature of the air fryer oven to 340ºF (171ºC). Press Start to begin preheating.

2. In a large bowl combine the onion, garlic, and gnocchi, and drizzle with the olive oil. Mix thoroughly.

3. Transfer the mixture to the air fryer oven and air fry for 15 minutes, stirring occasionally, making sure the gnocchi become light brown and crispy.

4. Add the pesto and Parmesan cheese, and give everything a good stir before serving.

Sriracha Golden Cauliflower

Prep time: 5 minutes | Cook time: 17 minutes | Serves 4

¼ cup vegan butter, melted

¼ cup sriracha sauce

4 cups cauliflower florets

1 cup bread crumbs

1 teaspoon salt

1. Set the temperature of the air fryer oven to 375ºF (191ºC). Press Start to begin preheating.
2. Mix the sriracha and vegan butter in a bowl and pour this mixture over the cauliflower, taking care to cover each floret entirely.
3. In a separate bowl, combine the bread crumbs and salt.
4. Dip the cauliflower florets in the bread crumbs, coating each one well. Air fry in the air fryer oven for 17 minutes.
5. Serve hot.

Sweet and Sour Tofu

Prep time: 15 minutes | Cook time: 20 minutes | Serves 2

2 teaspoons apple cider vinegar

1 tablespoon sugar

1 tablespoon soy sauce

3 teaspoons lime juice

1 teaspoon ground ginger

1 teaspoon garlic powder

½ block firm tofu, pressed to remove excess liquid and cut into cubes

1 teaspoon cornstarch

2 green onions, chopped

Toasted sesame seeds, for garnish

1. In a bowl, thoroughly combine the apple cider vinegar, sugar, soy sauce, lime juice, ground ginger, and garlic powder.

2. Cover the tofu with this mixture and leave to marinate for at least 30 minutes.

3. Set the temperature of the air fryer oven to 400ºF (204ºC). Press Start to begin preheating.

4. Transfer the tofu to the air fryer oven, keeping any excess marinade for the sauce. Air fry for 20 minutes or until crispy.

5. In the meantime, thicken the sauce with the cornstarch over a medium-low heat.

6. Serve the cooked tofu with the sauce, green onions, and sesame seeds.

Sweet Potato Fries

Prep time: 5 minutes | Cook time: 25 minutes | Serves 4

2 pounds (907 g) sweet potatoes, rinsed, sliced into matchsticks

1 teaspoon curry powder

2 tablespoons olive oil

Salt, to taste

1. Set the temperature of the air fryer oven to 390ºF (199ºC). Press Start to begin preheating.

2. Drizzle the oil in the perforated pan, place the fries inside and bake for 25 minutes.

3. Sprinkle with the curry powder and salt before serving.

Tofu Bites

Prep time: 15 minutes | Cook time: 30 minutes | Serves 4

1 packaged firm tofu, cubed and pressed to remove excess water

1 tablespoon soy sauce

1 tablespoon ketchup

1 tablespoon maple syrup

½ teaspoon vinegar

1 teaspoon liquid smoke

1 teaspoon hot sauce

2 tablespoons sesame seeds

1 teaspoon garlic powder

Salt and ground black pepper, to taste

Cooking spray

1. Set the temperature of the air fryer oven to 375ºF (191ºC). Press Start to begin preheating. Spritz the perforated pan with cooking spray.

2. Combine all the ingredients to coat the tofu completely and allow the marinade to absorb for half an hour.

3. Transfer the tofu to the pan, then air fry in the air fryer oven for 15 minutes. Flip the tofu over and air fry for another 15 minutes on the other side.

4. Serve immediately.

Zucchini Balls

Prep time: 5 minutes | Cook time: 10 minutes | Serves 4

4 zucchinis

1 egg

½ cup Parmesan cheese, grated

1 tablespoon Italian herbs

1 cup coconut, grated

1. Thinly grate the zucchini and dry with a cheesecloth, ensuring to remove all the moisture.

2. In a bowl, combine the zucchini with the egg, Parmesan, Italian herbs, and grated coconut, mixing well to incorporate everything. Using the hands, mold the mixture into balls.

3. Set the temperature of the air fryer oven to 400ºF (204ºC) and place the perforated pan inside. Press Start to begin preheating.

4. Lay the zucchini balls on the perforated pan and air fry for 10 minutes.

5. Serve hot.

Beef and Rice Stuffed Pepper

Prep time: 20 minutes | Cook time: 15 minutes | Serves 4

2 garlic cloves, minced

1 small onion, chopped

Cooking spray

1 pound (454 g) ground beef

1 teaspoon dried basil

½ teaspoon chili powder

1 teaspoon black pepper

1 teaspoon garlic salt

⅔ cup shredded cheese, divided

½ cup cooked rice

2 teaspoons Worcestershire sauce

8 ounces (227 g) tomato sauce

4 bell peppers, tops removed

1. Grease a frying pan with cooking spray and fry the onion and garlic over a medium heat.

2. Stir in the beef, basil, chili powder, black pepper, and garlic salt, combining everything well. Air fry until the beef is nicely browned, before taking the pan off the heat.

3. Add half of the cheese, the rice, Worcestershire sauce, and tomato sauce and stir to combine.

4. Spoon equal amounts of the beef mixture into the four bell peppers, filling them entirely.

5. Set the temperature of the air fryer oven to 400ºF (204ºC). Press Start to begin preheating.

6. Spritz the air fryer oven perforated pan with cooking spray.

7. Put the stuffed bell peppers in the perforated pan and air fry for 11 minutes.

8. Add the remaining cheese on top of each bell pepper and air fry for a further 2 minutes. When the cheese is melted and the bell peppers are piping hot, serve immediately.

Cashew Stuffed Mushrooms

Prep time: 10 minutes | Cook time: 15 minutes | Serves 6

1 cup basil

½ cup cashew, soaked overnight

½ cup nutritional yeast

1 tablespoon lemon juice

2 cloves garlic

1 tablespoon olive oil

Salt, to taste

1 pound (454 g) baby Bella mushroom, stems removed

1. Set the temperature of the air fryer oven to 400ºF (204ºC). Press Start to begin preheating.

2. Prepare the pesto. In a food processor, blend the basil, cashew nuts, nutritional yeast, lemon juice, garlic and olive oil to combine well. Sprinkle with salt as desired.

3. Turn the mushrooms cap-side down and spread the pesto on the underside of each cap.

4. Transfer to the air fryer oven and air fry for 15 minutes.

5. Serve warm.

Golden Garlicky Mushrooms

Prep time: 10 minutes | Cook time: 10 minutes | Serves 4

6 small mushrooms

1 tablespoon bread crumbs

1 tablespoon olive oil

1 ounce (28 g) onion, peeled and diced

1 teaspoon parsley

1 teaspoon garlic purée

Salt and ground black pepper, to taste

1. Set the temperature of the air fryer oven to 350ºF (177ºC). Press Start to begin preheating.

2. Combine the bread crumbs, oil, onion, parsley, salt, pepper and garlic in a bowl. Cut out the mushrooms' stalks and stuff each cap with the crumb mixture.

3. Air fry in the air fryer oven for 10 minutes.

4. Serve hot.

Gorgonzola Mushrooms with Horseradish Mayo

Prep time: 15 minutes | Cook time: 10 minutes | Serves 5

½ cup bread crumbs

2 cloves garlic, pressed

2 tablespoons chopped fresh coriander

⅓ teaspoon kosher salt

½ teaspoon crushed red pepper flakes

1½ tablespoons olive oil

20 medium mushrooms, stems removed

½ cup grated Gorgonzola cheese

¼ cup low-fat mayonnaise

1 teaspoon prepared horseradish, well-drained

1 tablespoon finely chopped fresh parsley

1. Set the temperature of the air fryer oven to 380ºF (193ºC). Press Start to begin preheating.

2. Combine the bread crumbs together with the garlic, coriander, salt, red pepper, and the olive oil.

3. Take equal-sized amounts of the bread crumb mixture and use them to stuff the mushroom caps. Add the grated Gorgonzola on top of each.

4. Put the mushrooms in the air fryer oven baking pan and transfer to the air fryer oven.

5. Air fry for 10 minutes, ensuring the stuffing is warm throughout.

6. In the meantime, prepare the horseradish mayo. Mix the mayonnaise, horseradish and parsley.

7. When the mushrooms are ready, serve with the mayo.

Kidney Beans Oatmeal in Peppers

Prep time: 15 minutes | Cook time: 6 minutes | Serves 2 to 4

2 large bell peppers, halved lengthwise, deseeded

2 tablespoons cooked kidney beans

2 tablespoons cooked chick peas

2 cups oatmeal, cooked

1 teaspoon ground cumin

½ teaspoon paprika

½ teaspoon salt or to taste

¼ teaspoon black pepper powder

¼ cup yogurt

1. Set the temperature of the air fryer oven to 355ºF (179ºC). Press Start to begin preheating.

2. Put the bell peppers, cut-side-down, in the air fryer oven. Air fry for 2 minutes.

3. Take the peppers out of the air fryer oven and let cool.

4. In a bowl, combine the rest of the ingredients.

5. Divide the mixture evenly and use each portion to stuff a pepper.

6. Return the stuffed peppers to the air fryer oven and continue to air fry for 4 minutes. Serve hot.

Jalapeño Poppers

Prep time: 5 minutes | Cook time: 33 minutes | Serves 4

8 medium jalapeño peppers

5 ounces (142 g) cream cheese

¼ cup grated Mozzarella cheese

½ teaspoon Italian seasoning mix

8 slices bacon

1. Set the temperature of the air fryer oven to 400ºF (204ºC). Press Start to begin preheating.

2. Cut the jalapeños in half.

3. Use a spoon to scrape out the insides of the peppers.

4. In a bowl, add together the cream cheese, Mozzarella cheese and Italian seasoning.

5. Pack the cream cheese mixture into the jalapeños halves and place the other halves on top.

6. Wrap each pepper in 1 slice of bacon, starting from the bottom and working up.

7. Bake for 33 minutes.

8. Serve immediately.

Marinara Pepperoni Mushroom Pizza

Prep time: 5 minutes | Cook time: 18 minutes | Serves 4

4 large portobello mushrooms, stems removed

4 teaspoons olive oil

1 cup marinara sauce

1 cup shredded Mozzarella cheese

10 slices sugar-free pepperoni

1. Set the temperature of the air fryer oven to 375ºF (191ºC). Press Start to begin preheating.

2. Brush each mushroom cap with the olive oil, one teaspoon for each cap.

3. Put on a baking sheet and bake stem side down for 8 minutes.

4. Take out of the air fryer oven and divide the marinara sauce, Mozzarella cheese and pepperoni evenly among the caps.

5. Air fry for another 10 minutes until browned.

6. Serve hot.

Prosciutto Mini Mushroom Pizza

Prep time: 10 minutes | Cook time: 5 minutes | Serves 3

3 portobello mushroom caps, cleaned and scooped

3 tablespoons olive oil

Pinch of salt

Pinch of dried Italian seasonings

3 tablespoons tomato sauce

3 tablespoons shredded Mozzarella cheese

12 slices prosciutto

1. Set the temperature of the air fryer oven to 330ºF (166ºC). Press Start to begin preheating.

2. Season both sides of the portobello mushrooms with a drizzle of olive oil, then sprinkle salt and the Italian seasonings on the insides.

3. With a knife, spread the tomato sauce evenly over the mushroom, before adding the Mozzarella on top.

4. Put the portobello in the perforated pan and place in the air fryer oven.

5. Air fry for 1 minute, before taking the perforated pan out of the air fryer oven and putting the prosciutto slices on top.

6. Air fry for another 4 minutes.

7. Serve warm.

Ricotta Potatoes

Prep time: 15 minutes | Cook time: 15 minutes | Serves 4

4 baking potatoes

2 tablespoons olive oil

½ cup Ricotta cheese, room temperature

2 tablespoons scallions, chopped

1 tablespoon fresh parsley, roughly chopped

1 tablespoon coriander, minced

2 ounces (57 g) Cheddar cheese, preferably freshly grated

1 teaspoon celery seeds

½ teaspoon salt

½ teaspoon garlic pepper

1. Set the temperature of the air fryer oven to 350ºF (177ºC). Press Start to begin preheating.

2. Pierce the skin of the potatoes with a knife.

3. Air fry in the air fryer oven perforated pan for 13 minutes. If they are not cooked through by this time, leave for 2 to 3 minutes longer.

4. In the meantime, make the stuffing by combining all the other ingredients.

5. Cut halfway into the cooked potatoes to open them.

6. Spoon equal amounts of the stuffing into each potato and serve hot.

Spicy Taco Stuffed Bell Peppers

Prep time: 10 minutes | Cook time: 30 minutes | Serves 4

1 pound (454 g) ground beef

1 tablespoon taco seasoning mix

1 can diced tomatoes and green chilis

4 green bell peppers

1 cup shredded Monterey jack cheese, divided

1. Set the temperature of the air fryer oven to 350ºF (177ºC). Press Start to begin preheating.

2. Set a skillet over a high heat and cook the ground beef for 8 minutes. Make sure it is cooked through and brown all over. Drain the fat.

3. Stir in the taco seasoning mix, and the diced tomatoes and green chilis. Allow the mixture to cook for a further 4 minutes.

4. In the meantime, slice the tops off the green peppers and remove the seeds and membranes.

5. When the meat mixture is fully cooked, spoon equal amounts of it into the peppers and top with the Monterey jack cheese. Then place the peppers into the air fryer oven. Air fry for 15 minutes.

6. The peppers are ready when they are soft, and the cheese is bubbling and brown. Serve warm.

Holiday Specials

Air Fried Spicy Olives

Prep time: 10 minutes | Cook time: 5 minutes | Serves 4

12 ounces (340 g) pitted black extra-large olives

¼ cup all-purpose flour

1 cup panko bread crumbs

2 teaspoons dried thyme

1 teaspoon red pepper flakes

1 teaspoon smoked paprika

1 egg beaten with 1 tablespoon water

Vegetable oil for spraying

1. Set the temperature of the air fryer oven to 400ºF (204ºC). Press Start to begin preheating.

2. Drain the olives and place them on a paper towel–lined plate to dry.

3. Put the flour on a plate. Combine the panko, thyme, red pepper flakes, and paprika on a separate plate. Dip an olive in the flour, shaking off any excess, then coat with egg mixture. Dredge the olive in the panko mixture, pressing to make the crumbs adhere, and place the breaded olive on a plate. Repeat with the remaining olives.

4. Spray the olives with oil and place them in a single layer in the air fryer oven perforated pan. Work in batches if necessary so as not to overcrowd the perforated pan. Air fry for 5 minutes until the breading is browned and crispy. Serve warm

Bourbon Monkey Bread

Prep time: 15 minutes | Cook time: 25 minutes | Serves 6 to 8

1 (16.3-ounce / 462-g) can store-bought refrigerated biscuit dough

¼ cup packed light brown sugar

1 teaspoon ground cinnamon

½ teaspoon freshly grated nutmeg

½ teaspoon ground ginger

½ teaspoon kosher salt

¼ teaspoon ground allspice

⅛ teaspoon ground cloves

4 tablespoons (½ stick) unsalted butter, melted

½ cup powdered sugar

2 teaspoons bourbon

2 tablespoons chopped candied cherries

2 tablespoons chopped pecans

1. Set the temperature of the air fryer oven to 310ºF (154ºC). Press Start to begin preheating.

2. Open the can and separate the biscuits, then cut each into quarters. Toss the biscuit quarters in a large bowl with the brown sugar, cinnamon, nutmeg, ginger, salt, allspice, and cloves until evenly coated. Transfer the dough pieces and any sugar left in the bowl to a cake pan, metal cake pan, or foil pan and drizzle evenly with the melted butter. Put the pan in the air fryer oven and bake until the monkey bread is golden brown and cooked through in the middle, about 25 minutes. Transfer the pan to a wire rack and let cool completely. Unmold from the pan.

3. In a small bowl, whisk the powdered sugar and the bourbon into a smooth glaze. Drizzle the glaze over the cooled monkey bread and, while the glaze is still wet, sprinkle with the cherries and pecans to serve.

Eggnog Bread

Prep time: 10 minutes | Cook time: 18 minutes | Serves 6 to 8

1 cup flour, plus more for dusting

¼ cup sugar

1 teaspoon baking powder

¼ teaspoon salt

¼ teaspoon nutmeg

½ cup eggnog

1 egg yolk

1 tablespoon plus 1 teaspoon butter, melted

¼ cup pecans

¼ cup chopped candied fruit (cherries, pineapple, or mixed fruits)

Cooking spray

1. Set the temperature of the air fryer oven to 360ºF (182ºC). Press Start to begin preheating.

2. In a medium bowl, stir together the flour, sugar, baking powder, salt, and nutmeg.

3. Add eggnog, egg yolk, and butter. Mix well but do not beat.

4. Stir in nuts and fruit.

5. Spray a baking pan with cooking spray and dust with flour.

6. Spread batter into prepared pan and bake for 18 minutes or until top is dark golden brown and bread starts to pull away from sides of pan.

7. Serve immediately.

Hasselback Potatoes

Prep time: 5 minutes | Cook time: 50 minutes | Serves 4

4 russet potatoes, peeled

Salt and freshly ground black pepper, to taste

¼ cup grated Parmesan cheese

Cooking spray

1. Set the temperature of the air fryer oven to 400ºF (204ºC). Press Start to begin preheating.

2. Spray the perforated pan lightly with cooking spray.

3. Make thin parallel cuts into each potato, ⅛-inch to ¼-inch apart, stopping at about ½ of the way through. The potato needs to stay intact along the bottom.

4. Spray the potatoes with cooking spray and use the hands or a silicone brush to completely coat the potatoes lightly in oil.

5. Put the potatoes, sliced side up, in the air fryer oven perforated pan in a single layer. Leave a little room between each potato. Sprinkle the potatoes lightly with salt and black pepper.

6. Air fry for 20 minutes. Reposition the potatoes and spritz lightly with cooking spray. Air fry until the potatoes are tender and crispy and browned, another 20 to 30 minutes.

7. Sprinkle the potatoes with Parmesan cheese and serve.

Hearty Honey Yeast Rolls

Prep time: 10 minutes | Cook time: 20 minutes | Makes 8 rolls

¼ cup whole milk, heated to 115ºF (46ºC) in the microwave

½ teaspoon active dry yeast

1 tablespoon honey

⅔ cup all-purpose flour, plus more for dusting

½ teaspoon kosher salt

2 tablespoons unsalted butter, at room temperature, plus more for greasing

Flaky sea salt, to taste

1. In a large bowl, whisk together the milk, yeast, and honey and let stand until foamy, about 10 minutes.

2. Stir in the flour and salt until just combined. Stir in the butter until absorbed. Scrape the dough onto a lightly floured work surface and knead until smooth, about 6 minutes. Transfer the dough to a lightly greased bowl, cover loosely with a sheet of plastic wrap or a kitchen towel, and let sit until nearly doubled in size, about 1 hour.

3. Uncover the dough, lightly press it down to expel the bubbles, then portion it into 8 equal pieces. Prepare the work surface by wiping it clean with a damp paper towel. Roll each piece into a ball by cupping the palm of the hand around the dough against the work surface and

moving the heel of the hand in a circular motion while using the thumb to contain the dough and tighten it into a perfectly round ball. Once all the balls are formed, nestle them side by side in the air fryer oven perforated pan.

4. Cover the rolls loosely with a kitchen towel or a sheet of plastic wrap and let sit until lightly risen and puffed, 20 to 30 minutes.

5. Set the temperature of the air fryer oven to 270ºF (132ºC). Press Start to begin preheating.

6. Uncover the rolls and gently brush with more butter, being careful not to press the rolls too hard. Air fry until the rolls are light golden brown and fluffy, about 12 minutes.

7. Remove the rolls from the air fryer oven and brush liberally with more butter, if you like, and sprinkle each roll with a pinch of sea salt. Serve warm.

Holiday Spicy Beef Roast

Prep time: 10 minutes | Cook time: 45 minutes | Serves 8

2 pounds (907 g) roast beef, at room temperature

2 tablespoons extra-virgin olive oil

1 teaspoon sea salt flakes

1 teaspoon black pepper, preferably freshly ground

1 teaspoon smoked paprika

A few dashes of liquid smoke

2 jalapeño peppers, thinly sliced

1. Set the temperature of the air fryer oven to 330ºF (166ºC). Press Start to begin preheating.

2. Pat the roast dry using kitchen towels. Rub with extra-virgin olive oil and all seasonings along with liquid smoke.

3. Roast for 30 minutes in the preheated air fryer oven. Turn the roast over and roast for additional 15 minutes.

4. Check for doneness using a meat thermometer and serve sprinkled with sliced jalapeños. Bon appétit!

Lush Snack Mix

Prep time: 10 minutes | Cook time: 10 minutes | Serves 10

½ cup honey

3 tablespoons butter, melted

1 teaspoon salt

2 cups sesame sticks

2 cup pumpkin seeds

2 cups granola

1 cup cashews

2 cups crispy corn puff cereal

2 cup mini pretzel crisps

1. In a bowl, combine the honey, butter, and salt.

2. In another bowl, mix the sesame sticks, pumpkin seeds, granola, cashews, corn puff cereal, and pretzel crisps.

3. Combine the contents of the two bowls.

4. Set the temperature of the air fryer oven to 370ºF (188ºC). Press Start to begin preheating.

5. Put the mixture in the air fryer oven perforated pan and air fry for 10 to 12 minutes to toast the snack mixture, shaking the perforated pan frequently. Do this in two batches.

6. Put the snack mix on a cookie sheet and allow it to cool fully.

7. Serve immediately.

Mushroom and Green Bean Casserole

Prep time: 10 minutes | Cook time: 15 minutes | Serves 4

4 tablespoons unsalted butter

¼ cup diced yellow onion

½ cup chopped white mushrooms

½ cup heavy whipping cream

1 ounce (28 g) full-fat cream cheese

½ cup chicken broth

¼ teaspoon xanthan gum

1 pound (454 g) fresh green beans, edges trimmed

½ ounce (14 g) pork rinds, finely ground

1. Set the temperature of the air fryer oven to 320ºF (160ºC). Press Start to begin preheating.

2. In a medium skillet over medium heat, melt the butter. Sauté the onion and mushrooms until they become soft and fragrant, about 3 to 5 minutes.

3. Add the heavy whipping cream, cream cheese, and broth. Whisk until smooth. Bring to a boil and then reduce to a simmer. Sprinkle the xanthan gum into the pan and remove from heat.

4. Chop the green beans into 2-inch pieces and place into a baking dish. Pour the sauce mixture over them and stir until coated. Top the dish with ground pork rinds. Put into the air fryer oven.

5. Adjust the temperature to 320ºF (160ºC) and set the timer for 15 minutes.

6. Top will be golden and green beans fork-tender when fully cooked. Serve warm.

Whole Chicken Roast

Prep time: 10 minutes | Cook time: 1 hour | Serves 6

1 teaspoon salt

1 teaspoon Italian seasoning

½ teaspoon freshly ground black pepper

½ teaspoon paprika

½ teaspoon garlic powder

½ teaspoon onion powder

2 tablespoons olive oil, plus more as needed

1 (4-pound / 1.8-kg) fryer chicken

1. Set the temperature of the air fryer oven to 360ºF (182ºC). Press Start to begin preheating.

2. Grease the perforated pan lightly with olive oil.

3. In a small bowl, mix the salt, Italian seasoning, pepper, paprika, garlic powder, and onion powder.

4. Remove any giblets from the chicken. Pat the chicken dry thoroughly with paper towels, including the cavity.

5. Brush the chicken all over with the olive oil and rub it with the seasoning mixture.

6. Truss the chicken or tie the legs with butcher's twine. This will make it easier to flip the chicken during cooking.

7. Put the chicken in the air fryer oven perforated pan, breast-side down. Air fry for 30 minutes. Flip the chicken over and baste it with any drippings collected in the bottom drawer of the air fryer oven. Lightly brush the chicken with olive oil.

8. Air fry for 20 minutes. Flip the chicken over one last time and air fry until a thermometer inserted into the thickest part of the thigh reaches at least 165ºF (74ºC) and it's crispy and golden, 10 more minutes. Continue to cook, checking every 5 minutes until the chicken reaches the correct internal temperature.

9. Let the chicken rest for 10 minutes before carving and serving.

CPSIA information can be obtained
at www.ICGtesting.com
Printed in the USA
LVHW021952010921
696703LV00014B/508

9 781802 909272